NATURE-BASED
SOCIAL PRESCRIBING

Integrating Nature-Based Interventions for Social and Environmental Wellbeing

A Handbook for Health Care Professionals

By

KIT KLINE

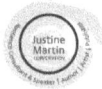

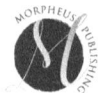

ISBN Paperback:	**978-1-7636985-8-1**
Author:	**Kit Kline**
Publisher:	**Justine Martin**
Editor:	**Justine Martin**
Artwork:	**Nathan Patterson**
Cover Graphics and Typesetting:	**Morpheus Publishing**

A catalogue record for this book is available from the **National Library of Australia**.

DISCLAIMER

The information contained in this book is for general informational purposes only. The author and publisher are not offering any medical, legal or professional advice. While every effort has been made to ensure the accuracy and completeness of the information provided, the author and publisher assume no responsibility for errors or omissions or any outcomes or consequences resulting from the use of this book's content.

DISTRIBUTION

This book is distributed by Morpheus Publishing and is available through authorised distributors, booksellers, Morpheus Publishing website and Kit Kline and www.https://www.naturebasedtherapy.com.au

COPYRIGHT PERMISSIONS

For copyright permissions or any other inquiries, please contact:

PUBLISHER: Morpheus Publishing
www.morpheuspublishing.com.au
hello@justinemartin.com.au
+61403 564 942

AUTHOR: Kit Kline
info@naturebasedtherapy.com.au
+61415 926 334
Wadawurrang Country
https://www.morpheuspublishing.com.au/authors/kit-kline

· Appendices ·

Table of Contents

· Appendices ·

Introduction

In today's fast-paced world, the connection between human well-being and nature has become more critical than ever. Nature-Based Social Prescribing (NBSP) provides an innovative and holistic approach to addressing social and environmental challenges. This handbook is designed to guide social workers in integrating nature-based interventions into their practice, fostering both individual and community well-being.

Chapter 1

Introduction to Nature-Based Social Prescribing

Overview:

Nature-Based Social Prescribing (NBSP) represents a growing movement in health and social care that harnesses the power of nature to support physical, mental, and social well-being. By connecting individuals to nature through personalised interventions, NBSP offers a holistic approach that addresses not only symptoms but also underlying social and environmental determinants of health. This chapter introduces the concept of NBSP, its relevance in contemporary social work, and the societal and environmental challenges that make it increasingly necessary.

Key Topics:

1.1 Definition and Principles of Nature-Based Social Prescribing

Nature-Based Social Prescribing (NBSP) refers to the practice of linking individuals to nature-related activities as part of their overall health and social care. It involves healthcare professionals, social workers, and community support organisations recommending and facilitating activities in natural environments to improve clients' well-being.

NBSP interventions can include activities such as nature walks, community gardening, conservation projects, outdoor mindfulness exercises, and more. These activities aim to improve physical health, reduce stress, increase social connections, and foster a deeper connection with the environment.

The principles of NBSP are rooted in a holistic view of health, recognizing the interconnection between individual well-being and the natural world. Key principles include:

- **Holistic Care:** Addressing the mental, emotional, physical, and social aspects of health.

- **Client-Centred:** Designing interventions that are tailored to the needs, preferences, and abilities of each individual.

- **Preventative and Therapeutic:** Using nature to both prevent illness and manage existing conditions.

- **Sustainability:** Promoting environmental stewardship alongside individual healing, encouraging sustainable relationships with the environment.

1.2 The Rise of Nature-Based Social Prescribing in Health and Social Care

The concept of prescribing nature has grown out of the recognition that the modern health and social care systems cannot address every aspect of well-being through traditional medical and psychological methods alone. The rise of NBSP is part of a broader trend emphasising non-clinical interventions, as seen in the growing fields of social prescribing and community-based health initiatives.

The roots of this approach can be traced to historical traditions of ecotherapy and outdoor-based healing practices used by Indigenous cultures around the world. In the last two decades, research has increasingly supported the idea that nature has profound therapeutic effects. As public health systems, particularly in countries like the UK and Australia, face growing pressures from an aging population, mental health crises, and environmental concerns, NBSP has emerged as an innovative solution to address these complex challenges.

Governments and health systems in various countries have recognised the benefits of nature-based interventions, leading to their inclusion in health and social care plans. This has also been influenced by growing public awareness of the need for sustainable living and the link between environmental health and human health.

1.3 Environmental and Social Factors Driving the Need for Nature-Based Social Prescribing

The need for NBSP is driven by both environmental and social factors, which are deeply interconnected. Many communities today face challenges related to:

- **Urbanisation:** Increasing urbanisation has reduced access to green spaces for many people. Large numbers of individuals live in cities where natural environments are limited or inaccessible, contributing to a sense of disconnection from nature.

- **Mental Health Crisis:** There is a rising prevalence of mental health issues globally, including anxiety, depression, and stress-related disorders. Nature-based interventions have been shown to reduce stress and improve mood, offering an accessible way to address these issues.

- **Social Isolation:** Many individuals, especially the elderly, feel socially isolated. Nature-based activities, particularly in group settings, can help foster community and reduce feelings of loneliness.

- **Climate Change and Environmental Degradation:** As the impacts of climate change become more pronounced, the need for solutions that foster resilience and adaptation is growing. NBSP can promote environmental stewardship, reconnect individuals to the land, and foster a more profound sense of responsibility toward sustainable living.

Social workers are uniquely positioned to address these factors due to their focus on supporting vulnerable populations, promoting social inclusion, and advocating for systemic change.

1.4 Benefits of Nature-Based Interventions for Physical, Mental, and Emotional Well-Being

There is substantial evidence that regular exposure to natural environments can significantly improve mental and physical health. Some key benefits of nature-based interventions include:

- **Improved Physical Health:** Activities such as gardening, hiking, and outdoor exercise promote physical fitness and reduce the risk of chronic conditions like cardiovascular disease, obesity, and diabetes.

- **Reduced Stress and Anxiety:** Nature has a calming effect on the mind, reducing levels of cortisol (the stress hormone) and promoting relaxation. Time spent in green spaces has been shown to lower blood pressure, improve sleep, and reduce symptoms of anxiety.

- **Enhanced Mood and Mental Clarity:** Exposure to nature has been linked to improvements in mood, increased feelings of happiness, and enhanced cognitive functioning. Natural environments offer a reprieve from the overstimulation of modern urban life, allowing individuals to reset and refresh.

- **Increased Social Interaction:** Many nature-based activities are conducted in group settings, promoting social interaction and reducing feelings of loneliness. Community gardening, for example, fosters cooperation, communication, and social bonds.

- **Connection to Something Greater:** Engaging with nature can create a sense of meaning and connection to something larger than oneself. This sense of awe and wonder is linked to positive mental health outcomes and increased feelings of purpose.

These benefits make NBSP an effective tool for addressing a wide range of issues, from physical ailments to mental health challenges, particularly in marginalised or underserved communities.

1.5 How NBSP Supports Holistic, Sustainable Care Approaches

NBSP aligns with the principles of holistic and sustainable care, offering a non-invasive, low-cost intervention that complements traditional social work practices. Social workers can use NBSP to address the whole person, recognising the interconnectedness of physical, emotional, mental, social, and environmental well-being.

Furthermore, NBSP encourages sustainable care practices by promoting environmental awareness and stewardship. In working with clients to foster their connection to nature, social workers can also engage them in environmental advocacy and conservation efforts, creating a positive feedback loop between individual health and environmental sustainability.

Conclusion: Nature-Based Social Prescribing offers an innovative, holistic approach that addresses the mental, emotional, and physical needs of clients while also promoting environmental stewardship. As you progress through this handbook, you will gain insights into the science, practical implementation, and evaluation of NBSP interventions, as well as the tools to integrate them effectively into your social work practice.

Case Study:

Clare, a 52-year-old woman, had been struggling with severe depression and social isolation for several years. After a series of failed attempts with traditional therapy, her social worker suggested trying a community gardening group as part of a Nature-Based Social Prescribing plan. At first, Clare was hesitant, feeling overwhelmed by the idea of socialising. However, over time, she found that working in the garden gave her a sense of calm and purpose. The simple act of planting and tending to flowers not only helped her feel more grounded, but also opened her up to new social connections. The gardening group became a lifeline, helping Clare regain confidence and a sense of community. Her depression symptoms lessened, and she became an advocate for green space initiatives in her local area.

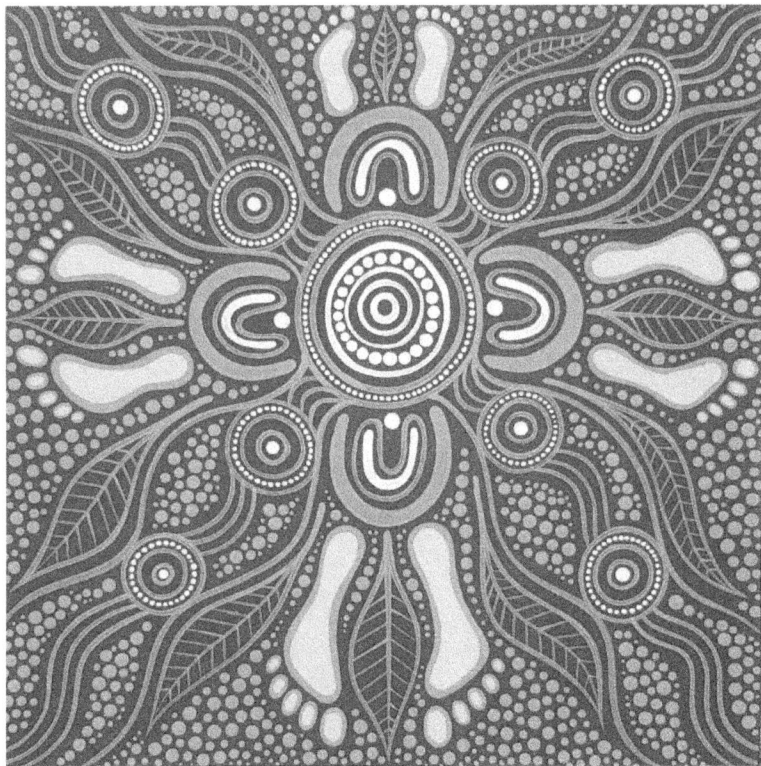

Bush Camp

Chapter 2

The Science Behind Nature-Based Interventions

Overview:

Nature-based interventions are supported by a growing body of scientific evidence that shows how interacting with nature can significantly improve mental, physical, and emotional well-being. This chapter explores the research and psychological theories that explain the therapeutic effects of nature. We will look at how the brain and body respond to natural environments, and how these responses translate into tangible health benefits. The chapter also introduces ecotherapy, the biophilia hypothesis, and the concept of "restorative environments" as frameworks that underpin the practice of Nature-Based Social Prescribing (NBSP).

Key Topics:

2.1 Overview of the Research on the Mental and Physical Health Benefits of Nature Exposure

The relationship between nature and human health has been the subject of extensive research across multiple disciplines, including psychology, neuroscience, and environmental science. Key studies over the last several decades have consistently shown that time spent in nature is associated with numerous health benefits. This section reviews some of the most important findings from the research literature.

- **Mental Health Benefits:** Numerous studies indicate that time spent in green spaces reduces symptoms of anxiety, depression, and stress. For instance, research conducted by Bratman et al. (2015) found that walking in nature significantly reduced rumination—a repetitive, negative thought pattern often associated with depression. Nature exposure has also been shown to improve mood, increase feelings of happiness, and enhance overall psychological well-being.

- **Physical Health Benefits:** Nature-based activities, such as hiking, gardening, and even simple walking, can improve cardiovascular health, reduce blood pressure, and enhance immune system function. One study by Li (2010) on the Japanese practice of "forest bathing" (Shinrin-Yoku) found that spending time in forests boosts the activity of natural killer (NK) cells, a component of the immune system that helps fight off infections and cancer.

- **Cognitive Function:** Research by Berman et al. (2008) demonstrated that exposure to natural environments improves cognitive function, particularly attention and memory. This is linked to the "Attention Restoration Theory," which suggests that natural environments engage the brain in a way that allows for cognitive recovery and improved focus.

- **Social Connection:** Being in nature, especially in group settings, fosters social connection and a sense of community. Research by Holt-Lunstad et al. (2010) has demonstrated that social isolation is a significant risk factor for mortality, highlighting the importance of social connection in overall well-being.

2.2 Ecotherapy and Its Foundations in Mental Health Care

Ecotherapy, also known as nature-based therapy or green therapy, is a therapeutic practice that emphasises the healing power of nature. It is based on the premise that humans have an inherent need to connect with the natural world and that this connection promotes healing, growth, and well-being. Ecotherapy encompasses a wide range of nature-based interventions, from walking in nature to more structured activities like horticultural therapy or wilderness therapy.

Key Components of Ecotherapy:

- **Connection with Nature:** Ecotherapy focuses on fostering a deep connection between individuals and the natural world. This connection is thought to help individuals develop a sense of meaning and belonging, which can be particularly beneficial for those struggling with feelings of isolation or alienation.

- **Mindfulness in Nature:** Many ecotherapy practices incorporate mindfulness techniques, encouraging individuals to engage their senses fully in the present moment while in natural settings. This promotes relaxation and stress reduction, as well as a heightened awareness of one's surroundings and internal states.

- **Therapeutic Alliance:** In ecotherapy, the relationship between therapist and client is important, but nature itself is also considered a co-therapist. The natural environment serves as a healing space that can facilitate emotional and psychological breakthroughs.

- **Supporting Research:** Research by Jordan and Hinds (2016) highlights that ecotherapy interventions can reduce symptoms of depression, anxiety, and stress, while also promoting personal growth and positive environmental attitudes. Studies have found that patients with depression who participated in outdoor group activities, such as gardening or walking in nature, showed significant improvements in their mood and self-esteem compared to control groups.

2.3 The Biophilia Hypothesis: Human Beings' Innate Connection to Nature

The Biophilia Hypothesis, popularized by biologist E.O. Wilson, suggests that humans have an innate affinity for nature and natural processes. According to this theory, our evolutionary history as a species that lived closely with nature for thousands of years has shaped our brains and bodies to respond positively to natural environments.

Core Concepts of Biophilia:

- **Innate Preference:** Humans are naturally drawn to certain elements of the natural world, such as trees, water, and open landscapes, because these environments historically provided food, shelter, and safety.

- **Emotional Responses:** Natural environments elicit positive emotional responses, such as feelings of calm, awe, and wonder. These emotions are linked to mental health benefits, including reduced stress and improved mood.

- **Health and Well-Being:** Biophilic environments can improve mental and physical health by reducing stress and promoting relaxation. The presence of green spaces in urban areas, for example, has been associated with lower levels of crime and improved community well-being (Ulrich, 1984).

The biophilia hypothesis provides a theoretical foundation for Nature-Based Social Prescribing by explaining why natural environments are so effective at promoting health and well-being. It also reinforces the idea that reconnecting with nature is not just a luxury but a fundamental human need.

2.4 The Role of Natural Environments in Reducing Stress, Anxiety, and Depression

One of the most well-documented benefits of spending time in nature is its ability to reduce stress. Studies have shown that being in nature lowers levels of cortisol, the hormone associated with stress and increases feelings of relaxation and calm. Natural environments are thought to provide a "soft fascination" that captures attention without overwhelming the mind, allowing for cognitive recovery and emotional regulation.

- **Stress Reduction:** Ulrich's (1991) Stress Recovery Theory suggests that natural environments facilitate quick recovery from stress by reducing autonomic arousal (such as heart rate and blood pressure) and restoring emotional balance. This is particularly relevant for social workers who work with clients experiencing high levels of stress or trauma.

- **Anxiety and Depression:** Research by Martyn and Brymer (2016) has shown that nature-based interventions can alleviate symptoms of anxiety and depression by providing a space for reflection, mindfulness, and emotional processing. The natural world offers a non-judgmental and soothing environment that can help individuals work through difficult emotions.

- **Physical Activity in Nature:** Physical activities such as hiking, cycling, or even walking in nature amplify the benefits of stress reduction and mental well-being. Green exercise, a term coined to describe physical activity in natural environments, has been shown to improve mood, self-esteem, and cognitive function (Pretty et al., 2005).

2.5 Evidence from Studies on Forest Bathing, Green Exercise, and Horticultural Therapy

Forest Bathing (Shinrin-Yoku): Originating in Japan, forest bathing involves immersing oneself in the forest atmosphere and mindfully engaging with nature through the senses. A 2010 study by Li and colleagues found that forest bathing significantly lowers cortisol levels, reduces blood pressure, and enhances immune system function. It has been adopted worldwide as an effective intervention for reducing stress and promoting mental health.

Green Exercise: Engaging in physical activity in natural settings, such as walking in a park or jogging by a lake, has been shown to have added benefits compared to indoor exercise. Research by Pretty et al. (2005) suggests that even brief exposure to green spaces while exercising can lead to improvements in self-esteem and mood.

Horticultural Therapy: Gardening has long been recognised as a therapeutic activity, particularly for individuals dealing with mental health challenges, trauma, or social isolation. Horticultural therapy involves working with plants and natural elements to promote physical and emotional well-being. Research by Gonzalez et al. (2010) showed that horticultural therapy improves mood, reduces symptoms of depression, and increases feelings of accomplishment and self-efficacy.

Conclusion:

The scientific evidence supporting Nature-Based Social Prescribing is robust, with numerous studies demonstrating its effectiveness in promoting mental, physical, and emotional well-being. Understanding the science behind these interventions provides social workers with the knowledge and confidence to integrate NBSP into their practice, offering clients a powerful tool for holistic healing.

Practical Tool: Breathing Exercise for Clients

When engaging in nature-based interventions, mindfulness practices can enhance the therapeutic benefits of nature. Here is a simple breathing exercise to use during outdoor sessions:

1. **Find a comfortable spot:** Whether sitting or standing, make sure you are comfortable and can observe your surroundings.

2. **Engage your senses:** Close your eyes and take a moment to feel the air on your skin, hear the sounds of nature around you, and smell the natural scents.

3. **Breathe deeply:** Inhale slowly through your nose for a count of four, hold your breath for a count of four, and then exhale through your mouth for a count of four.

4. **Repeat:** Continue this deep, mindful breathing for several minutes, allowing yourself to relax and connect with the environment.

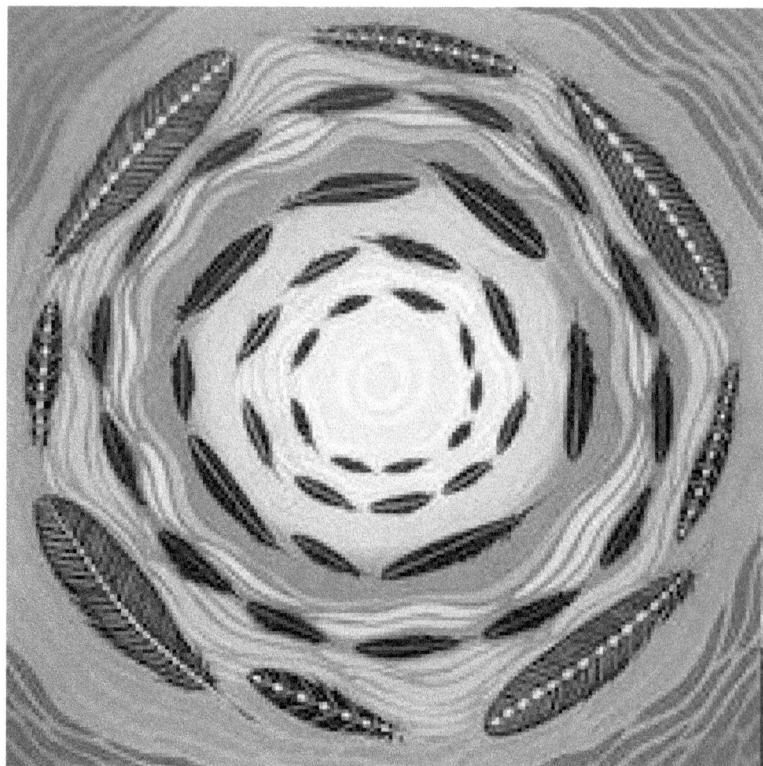

Leaves

Chapter 3

Integrating Nature-Based Prescribing into Social Work Practice

Overview:

Nature-Based Social Prescribing (NBSP) holds tremendous potential for social workers seeking to offer holistic, non-clinical interventions that address clients' mental, physical, and social well-being. In this chapter, we focus on the practical aspects of incorporating NBSP into social work, including understanding the referral process, designing appropriate interventions, assessing client readiness, and navigating potential challenges. The chapter also explores how social workers can collaborate with community organizations to create sustainable and accessible nature-based interventions.

Key Topics:

3.1 The Role of Social Workers in Facilitating Nature-Based Interventions

Social workers play a pivotal role in facilitating NBSP interventions. Their unique position as advocates, facilitators, and support providers enables them to connect clients to nature-based activities that promote health and well-being. Social workers often deal with complex cases involving trauma, mental health issues, and social isolation—challenges that nature-based interventions are particularly well-suited to address.

Social workers can integrate NBSP by:

- **Assessing client needs:** Identifying clients who may benefit from NBSP interventions based on their physical, mental, emotional, and social needs.

- **Collaborating with healthcare professionals:** Partnering with GPs, psychologists, and other healthcare providers to ensure a comprehensive approach to care that includes nature-based interventions.

- **Designing personalized interventions:** Working with clients to co-create tailored nature-based activities that align with their goals, preferences, and abilities.

- **Advocating for access to nature:** Social workers can advocate for increased access to green spaces, parks, and community gardens, particularly for marginalized populations.

Social workers are also responsible for ensuring that interventions are inclusive and accessible, considering factors such as mobility, cultural relevance, and environmental barriers.

3.2 Designing Individualised Nature-Based Prescribing Plans

Individualized prescribing plans are at the heart of effective NBSP. Every client has unique circumstances, so it's essential that interventions are tailored to their specific needs, preferences, and capabilities. The goal is to provide activities that are not only therapeutic but also enjoyable and sustainable for the client.

Steps to Design an Individualized NBSP Plan:

- **Initial Assessment:** During the assessment phase, the social worker should gather detailed information about the client's physical and mental health, lifestyle, interests, and barriers to participating in nature-based activities. Understanding the client's comfort level with nature and their previous experiences (if any) will help in creating a relevant plan.

- **Co-Creation with the Client:** A client-centred approach is key. Clients should have input in selecting activities that align with their preferences. For instance, some may enjoy the tranquillity of a park, while others may prefer the social aspect of community gardening.

- **Goal Setting:** Establishing clear goals for the intervention is important for tracking progress and ensuring that the activity remains purposeful. Goals may include reducing stress, improving social connections, increasing physical activity, or boosting self-esteem.

- **Activity Selection:** The activities chosen should be manageable and enjoyable for the client. Examples of activities include nature walks, gardening, forest bathing, bird watching, outdoor yoga, and beach clean-ups.

- **Logistics and Support:** Social workers should ensure that the logistics are in place, such as transportation to natural settings, access to appropriate clothing or equipment, and safety considerations. It's also crucial to assess whether the client needs support during the activities, such as guidance from a therapist or peer support.

Example: John, a 45-year-old recovering from substance abuse, expressed an interest in nature but had no previous experience with outdoor activities. His social worker created a plan that began with short nature walks in a local park, gradually introducing him to more immersive activities such as joining a community gardening project. Over time, John found that these activities helped him manage stress and build a support network, contributing to his recovery journey.

3.3 Assessing Client Readiness and Capacity for Nature-Based Activities

Not all clients are immediately ready or willing to engage in nature-based activities, and it's essential for social workers to assess their readiness. Readiness can depend on various factors, including physical health, emotional well-being, motivation, and familiarity with nature.

Assessing Client Readiness:

Social workers can use tools such as the Stages of Change Model to gauge where clients are in terms of readiness:

- **Pre-contemplation:** Clients may be unaware of the benefits of NBSP or may not believe it will help them.

- **Contemplation:** Clients recognize the potential benefits of NBSP but may still be ambivalent.

- **Preparation:** Clients are ready to engage in nature-based activities and may need support to take the first step.

- **Action:** Clients actively participate in NBSP activities.

- **Maintenance:** Clients have integrated NBSP into their regular routines and continue to benefit from it.

Assessing capacity also includes physical limitations (such as mobility issues), mental health considerations (such as anxiety about being in open spaces), and practical barriers (such as access to transportation). The goal is to meet the client where they are and gradually increase their engagement with nature-based interventions.

3.4 Overcoming Barriers to Nature-Based Social Prescribing

While NBSP offers many benefits, there are challenges in implementing these interventions, particularly for clients who may face barriers to accessing natural environments. Social workers must be adept at identifying and overcoming these barriers to ensure that all clients can benefit from NBSP.

Common Barriers and Solutions:

- **Accessibility:** Clients with physical disabilities or limited mobility may find it challenging to participate in outdoor activities. Solutions may include identifying accessible parks, wheelchair-friendly trails, or urban green spaces that are designed for inclusivity.

- **Geographical Barriers:** In some urban areas, green spaces may be limited or difficult to access. Social workers can collaborate with community organizations to create nature-based activities in local parks, rooftops, or community gardens, bringing nature to urban settings.

- **Cultural and Emotional Barriers:** Some clients may not feel comfortable in natural environments, either due to unfamiliarity or cultural perceptions. In these cases, social workers should be sensitive to clients' backgrounds and preferences, offering gradual exposure or culturally relevant activities.

- **Logistical Barriers:** Transportation, time constraints, and financial resources can limit access to nature-based interventions. Social workers can partner with local organizations that provide transportation, equipment, or free access to nature-based programs.

Example: Maria, a 65-year-old with limited mobility, was interested in nature but found it difficult to visit local parks. Her social worker collaborated with a community organization that provided wheelchair-accessible garden plots, enabling

Maria to participate in horticultural therapy from her home. This small but meaningful change gave her a sense of purpose and connection with nature, despite her mobility challenges.

3.5 Collaborating with Community Partners and Organisations

Collaboration with community partners is key to the successful implementation of NBSP. Social workers are often the bridge between clients and local organizations that can provide nature-based programs, such as parks and recreation departments, environmental organizations, and health clinics.

Building Partnerships:

Social workers can:

- **Engage local parks and nature reserves:** Many parks offer programs such as guided nature walks, outdoor fitness classes, or conservation projects that can be incorporated into NBSP.

- **Collaborate with community gardens:** Community gardens offer clients the opportunity to engage in horticultural therapy, grow their own food, and connect with others.

- **Partner with environmental NGOs:** Environmental organizations often run volunteer programs or eco-restoration projects that clients can participate in, helping them connect with nature while contributing to conservation efforts.

Creating Referral Pathways:

To ensure clients can access nature-based interventions, social workers should establish clear referral pathways with local organizations. This may involve formal partnerships with community health centers, outdoor therapy providers, or nature-based non-profits that specialize in offering accessible and inclusive nature programs.

Example: Through collaboration with a local environmental group, a social worker created a pathway for at-risk youth to participate in a reforestation project. The project provided therapeutic benefits for the youth while also teaching them valuable skills and environmental stewardship. The partnership proved to be mutually beneficial for both the clients and the community.

3.6 Embedding Nature-Based Prescribing into Organizational Practice

For NBSP to be successful, it must be embedded into the broader practice of social work organizations. This requires organizational commitment, training, and resources to support social workers in implementing these interventions.

Social work agencies can incorporate NBSP into their practice by:

- **Training staff:** Providing social workers with the knowledge and skills to design and facilitate nature-based interventions.

- **Developing protocols:** Creating protocols for referring clients to NBSP and ensuring that interventions are tracked and evaluated.

- **Allocating resources:** Supporting initiatives that provide clients with access to natural environments, such as partnering with local parks or offering transportation to nature-based activities.

By embedding NBSP into their organizational practice, social work agencies can create sustainable, long-term interventions that benefit both clients and the community.

Conclusion:

Integrating Nature-Based Social Prescribing into social work practice requires thoughtful planning, collaboration, and a client-centred approach. Social workers can play a vital role in designing and facilitating interventions that harness the power of nature to support holistic health and well-being. By overcoming barriers, collaborating with community partners, and embedding NBSP into organisational practice, social workers can create sustainable and impactful interventions for their clients.

Practical Tool: Nature Walk Reflection

After completing a nature walk with a client, encourage them to reflect on their experience using the following prompts:

1. What did you notice during the walk? Focus on sounds, smells, or sights.

2. How did the environment make you feel?

3. Did you notice any changes in your mood or thoughts during or after the walk?

4. What aspects of the walk would you like to explore more in the future?

Chapter 4

Understanding the Benefits of Nature-Based Social Prescribing

Overview:

This chapter explores the diverse benefits of Nature-Based Social Prescribing (NBSP) for mental, physical, social, and environmental well-being. Backed by research, NBSP has been shown to support improvements in mental health, promote social connection, and foster physical wellness. In addition, engaging with nature encourages environmental stewardship and a deeper sense of connection to the earth. This chapter discusses each of these benefits in detail and provides practical examples of how they manifest in clients' lives.

Key Topics:

4.1 Mental Health Benefits

Nature has a profound impact on mental health, offering a respite from the stressors of modern life and providing opportunities for mindfulness, reflection, and emotional healing. NBSP can be particularly beneficial for clients dealing with anxiety, depression, trauma, and stress, offering a natural and accessible way to promote mental well-being.

Specific Mental Health Benefits of NBSP:

- **Stress Reduction:** Time in nature has been shown to reduce cortisol levels and lower blood pressure, providing immediate relief from stress.

- **Improved Mood:** Regular exposure to nature can increase the production of serotonin, improving mood and combating feelings of depression.

- **Enhanced Focus and Attention:** Natural environments have been found to help restore attention and reduce symptoms of ADHD, allowing clients to focus better and process emotions.

- **Mindfulness and Grounding:** Nature-based activities like walking or gardening encourage mindfulness, helping clients stay present and grounded, which can alleviate anxiety.

Example: Sarah, a client dealing with anxiety and work-related stress, participated in weekly forest therapy sessions. She found that being in nature helped her slow down, breathe deeply, and reduce her anxious thoughts.

Over time, she reported feeling calmer and better able to manage her daily stressors.

4.2 Physical Health Benefits

Engaging in nature-based activities also contributes to physical health, offering a low-cost, accessible way to incorporate movement and exercise into daily life. Activities like walking, gardening, hiking, and even swimming in natural bodies of water provide cardiovascular benefits, increase strength and flexibility, and improve overall physical health.

Specific Physical Health Benefits of NBSP:

- **Increased Physical Activity:** Nature-based interventions encourage physical movement, which can improve cardiovascular health, support weight management, and reduce the risk of chronic illnesses such as diabetes and heart disease.

- **Improved Sleep:** Regular exposure to natural light and outdoor environments can help regulate sleep patterns, which is particularly helpful for clients struggling with insomnia.

- **Boosted Immune System:** Time spent outdoors, especially in green environments, has been shown to boost the immune system, supporting the body's natural defences against illness.

- **Pain Reduction:** Studies have found that engaging with nature can reduce the perception of pain and improve overall well-being for clients with chronic pain conditions.

Example: Tom, a 60-year-old client with chronic back pain, was prescribed a nature-based intervention involving weekly walks along a forest trail. He found that walking in nature not only helped alleviate his pain but also boosted his mood and provided an opportunity for gentle exercise that felt accessible and enjoyable.

4.3 Social Benefits

NBSP offers unique opportunities for clients to foster social connections, particularly for those who may feel isolated or disconnected. Whether through community gardening projects, group nature walks, or volunteer environmental programs, nature-based activities encourage social interaction and the development of meaningful relationships.

Specific Social Benefits of NBSP:

- **Building Social Connections:** Group activities in nature create opportunities for clients to build relationships, reducing feelings of isolation and loneliness.

- **Community Engagement:** Participating in community-based nature activities, such as urban farming or neighbourhood clean-up events, fosters a sense of belonging and contributes to the community.

- **Support Networks:** Nature-based interventions can also help clients develop support networks, as they bond with others over shared experiences in natural settings.

Example: A group of older adults at a social work centre was prescribed a community gardening project. Over the course of several months, the group formed close bonds, sharing stories while tending the garden. Many reported that this project gave them a renewed sense of purpose and connection, reducing feelings of loneliness.

4.4 Environmental Benefits and Stewardship

In addition to benefiting individual clients, NBSP promotes environmental stewardship by encouraging people to engage with and care for natural spaces. When clients participate in nature-based activities, they often develop a deeper connection to the environment, which fosters a sense of responsibility for protecting the earth.

Specific Environmental Benefits of NBSP:

- **Encouraging Sustainability:** Clients who engage in nature-based activities often develop a greater appreciation for the environment and are more likely to adopt sustainable practices in their daily lives.

- **Promoting Conservation:** NBSP can connect clients with environmental conservation projects, such as tree planting, habitat restoration, or beach clean-ups, giving them an opportunity to contribute positively to the environment.

- **Fostering Environmental Awareness:** Engaging in nature helps clients develop an awareness of local ecosystems and the impact of human activity on the planet, fostering long-term environmental responsibility.

Example: When Jack joined a local reforestation project as part of his NBSP plan, he not only improved his mental and physical health but also became passionate about environmental conservation. He continued volunteering with the project, helping plant trees and educate others on the importance of protecting natural ecosystems.

4.5 Holistic Well-Being: Connecting Mental, Physical, Social, and Environmental Health

NBSP's strength lies in its ability to address the full spectrum of well-being, offering an integrated approach that connects mental, physical, social, and environmental health. By engaging with nature, clients experience holistic benefits that contribute to overall well-being.

Integrating Well-Being into Practice:

Social workers should emphasize the interconnectedness of these benefits when prescribing nature-based interventions. Clients who start with a nature walk to reduce stress may soon discover physical improvements, enhanced social connections, and a growing awareness of their relationship with the environment.

Conclusion:

The benefits of Nature-Based Social Prescribing are far-reaching, offering holistic improvements to clients' mental, physical, social, and environmental well-being. By understanding and emphasizing these benefits, social workers can confidently prescribe nature-based interventions as part of a comprehensive care plan, knowing that the positive effects will extend beyond individual health to foster community engagement and environmental stewardship.

Practical Tool: Reflection on Nature's Impact

Encourage clients to journal after participating in a nature-based activity, reflecting on how the experience has impacted their mental, physical, social, and environmental well-being. Prompts might include:

1. How did your mood change after the activity?

2. Did you notice any physical sensations, like increased energy or relaxation?

3. How did the activity influence your sense of connection to others or the environment?

4. What aspects of the experience would you like to continue exploring?

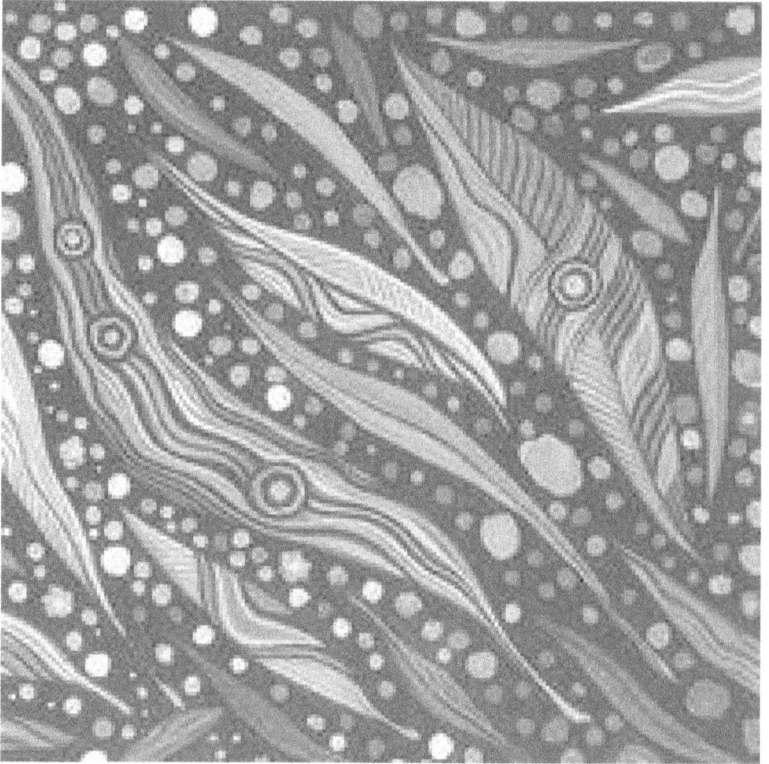

Nature 2

Chapter 5

Evaluating Nature-Based Interventions

Overview:

Evaluation is a crucial component of any intervention, and Nature-Based Social Prescribing is no different. This chapter focuses on methods for evaluating the effectiveness of NBSP interventions, including qualitative and quantitative approaches, client feedback, and long-term outcomes. Social workers will learn how to assess the impact of nature-based interventions on clients' mental, physical, social, and environmental well-being and make adjustments as needed.

Key Topics:

5.1 Why Evaluate Nature-Based Interventions?

Evaluating the effectiveness of NBSP interventions helps ensure that they are meeting the needs of clients and achieving the intended outcomes. It also provides evidence for the value of nature-based interventions, which can support funding applications, partnerships with community organizations, and the integration of NBSP into broader healthcare systems.

Social workers need to evaluate interventions to:

- **Measure Client Progress:** Determine whether clients are achieving their health and well-being goals through the prescribed activities.

- **Ensure Quality:** Make sure that the nature-based interventions are effective, accessible, and appropriate for each client.

- **Refine Practice:** Use evaluation data to adjust interventions, refine techniques, and explore new opportunities for integrating nature-based approaches into social work practice.

5.2 Quantitative Evaluation Tools

Quantitative tools provide measurable data on the effectiveness of NBSP interventions. These tools may assess physical health improvements, psychological changes, and social engagement.

Examples of Quantitative Evaluation Tools:

- **Surveys and Questionnaires:** Clients can complete standardized surveys before and after the intervention to measure changes in mood, stress levels, physical activity, or social engagement.

- **Biometric Measures:** In some cases, social workers may collaborate with healthcare providers to assess biometric indicators such as blood pressure, heart rate, or cortisol levels before and after nature-based activities.

- **Activity Logs:** Clients can track their participation in nature-based activities and note any changes in mood, energy levels, or social interactions.

Example: A group of clients participating in a gardening project completed the Perceived Stress Scale (PSS) at the beginning and end of a 12-week program. The results showed a significant decrease in stress levels, demonstrating the effectiveness of the intervention.

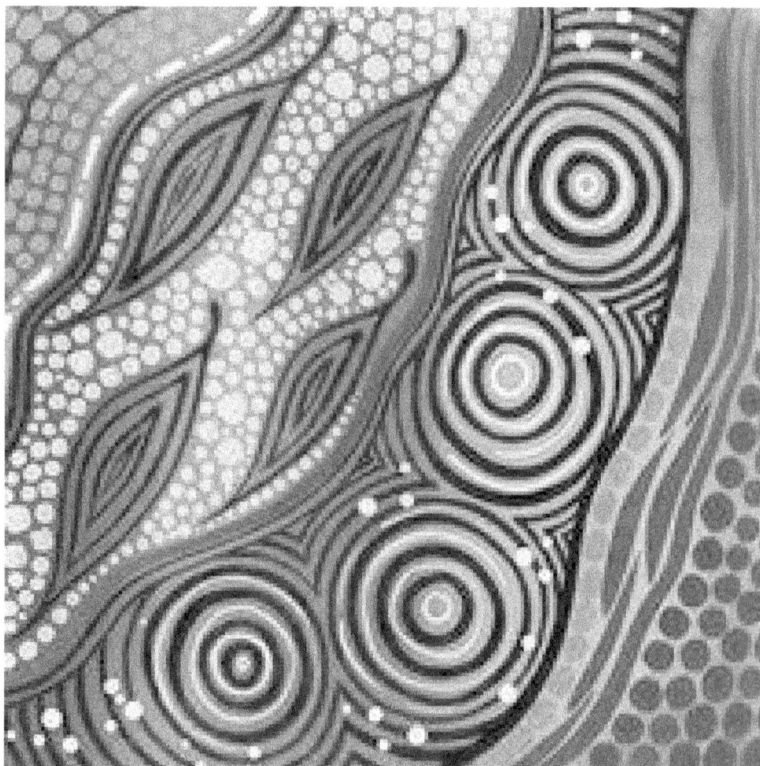

Nature

Chapter 6

Addressing Challenges in Implementing Nature-Based Social Prescribing

Overview:

While the benefits of Nature-Based Social Prescribing (NBSP) are numerous, there are also challenges to implementing it in practice. Social workers may encounter logistical, environmental, financial, or cultural barriers that prevent the seamless integration of nature-based interventions into client care. This chapter explores common challenges and offers strategies for overcoming them, ensuring that NBSP can be effectively delivered to a wide range of clients.

Key Topics:

6.1 Logistical Challenges

Practical concerns like access to nature, time constraints, and transportation issues can limit clients' ability to engage in NBSP. Some clients may live in urban areas with limited access to green spaces, or they may face physical or mobility challenges that make outdoor activities difficult.

Strategies to Overcome Logistical Challenges:

- **Creative Use of Urban Green Spaces:** Even in densely populated urban areas, there are opportunities for nature-based interventions. Rooftop gardens, urban parks, community green spaces, and even indoor nature therapy through potted plants or greenhouses can provide an accessible option for clients.

- **Flexible Scheduling**: Many clients have busy schedules that make it hard to commit to regular outdoor activities. Social workers can recommend short, daily practices such as mindful walks during lunch breaks or simply sitting outside for a few minutes to connect with nature.

- **Digital Nature Prescriptions:** For clients with severe mobility issues or living in areas without accessible nature, technology can provide an alternative. Virtual nature experiences through apps, guided meditation videos featuring natural environments, or even soundscapes of birds, rivers, or forests can evoke similar benefits to physical immersion in nature.

Example: Jane, a client in a wheelchair, was unable to access local hiking trails, but her social worker prescribed a daily 10-minute practice of listening to ocean sounds while sitting near her apartment window. This practice helped reduce her stress and improved her overall well-being.

6.2 Environmental and Seasonal Considerations

Nature-based interventions depend on the natural environment, which can present challenges in areas affected by extreme weather, seasonal changes, or environmental degradation. Clients living in areas prone to harsh winters or extreme heat may have difficulty engaging in outdoor activities during certain times of the year.

Strategies to Overcome Environmental Challenges:

- **Seasonal Adaptation:** Social workers can develop seasonal plans for clients, with indoor nature-based activities like houseplant care or nature journaling during the winter, and outdoor activities during milder months.

- **Use of Shelter and Shaded Areas:** For clients in hot climates, social workers can recommend engaging in nature-based activities in shaded parks or community gardens, where there is shelter from the sun.

- **Environmental Advocacy:** When nature is threatened by urban development or environmental degradation, NBSP programs can encourage clients to become advocates for local green spaces, connecting personal well-being with environmental activism.

Example: A social worker in a region with harsh winters developed a winter nature-care plan for clients that included indoor gardening, birdwatching from windows, and nature-inspired crafts, helping clients stay connected to nature year-round.

6.3 Financial Barriers

Nature-based interventions can often be low-cost or free, but some clients may still face financial barriers, particularly if specialized equipment, transportation, or access fees to parks and reserves are involved.

Strategies to Overcome Financial Barriers:

- **Low-Cost and Free Activities:** Social workers can guide clients to free or low-cost nature activities such as visiting local parks, walking trails, or community gardens. Additionally, encouraging activities like foraging or using nature's materials for crafts (e.g., rock painting) can provide affordable ways to engage with nature.

- **Partnerships and Funding:** Social workers can also collaborate with local environmental organizations, outdoor activity groups, or parks services to secure free or discounted access to nature-based programs. In some cases, grants or government funding can be accessed to support clients in need.

Example: Tom, a client facing financial difficulties, was interested in hiking but could not afford transportation to a nearby nature reserve. His social worker partnered with a local outdoor club that offered free weekend transportation for community members.

6.4 Cultural and Individual Preferences

Not all clients may feel comfortable or motivated to engage in nature-based activities, particularly if their cultural background or personal experiences have shaped different views on nature. Some may feel disconnected from nature, or even fear certain natural environments, such as forests or bodies of water.

Strategies to Overcome Cultural and Personal Barriers:

- **Personalised Interventions:** Social workers should take the time to understand each client's cultural background, personal history, and individual preferences. Instead of prescribing a one-size-fits-all nature experience, they can co-create personalized plans that reflect the client's comfort level with nature.

- **Culturally Relevant Practices:** Some clients may resonate more with culturally specific nature-based practices, such as Indigenous approaches to nature, storytelling, or rituals that connect them to their ancestry. Social workers should be mindful of integrating culturally respectful and relevant practices into NBSP.

- **Gradual Exposure:** For clients who may feel fearful or disconnected from nature, starting with smaller, controlled activities—such as simply sitting outside or planting a small herb garden—can help them slowly build a positive relationship with nature.

Example: Maria, a client with a fear of water, was hesitant to join a group canoeing activity. Her social worker recommended starting with a nature walk along a stream to gently reintroduce her to natural bodies of water, gradually helping her become more comfortable.

6.5 Institutional and Policy-Level Barriers

Implementing NBSP at a larger, institutional level can face challenges such as lack of funding, resistance from traditional healthcare models, or a lack of awareness among stakeholders about the benefits of NBSP.

Strategies to Overcome Institutional Barriers:

- **Education and Advocacy:** Social workers can advocate for NBSP by educating colleagues, healthcare providers, and policymakers about the proven benefits of nature-based interventions. Presenting research data and client success stories can help garner institutional support.

- **Developing Collaborative Partnerships:** Collaborating with environmental organizations, government agencies, or public health departments can create a network of support for integrating NBSP into mainstream care.

- **Policy Change:** At a higher level, social workers can get involved in policy advocacy to push for government funding, environmental conservation, and the formal recognition of NBSP within healthcare systems.

Example: A social worker successfully lobbied for a partnership between the local health department and a nearby nature preserve, resulting in a program where clients could access free nature-based therapy sessions with the support of local government funding.

Practical Tool: Barrier Identification Worksheet

Use this worksheet with clients to identify potential barriers to engaging with nature-based interventions and explore possible solutions.

1. What practical challenges do you face when accessing nature (e.g., time, transportation, mobility)?

2. Are there any environmental concerns (e.g., weather, safety, pollution) that might limit your participation?

3. What financial resources, if any, are needed for you to participate in nature-based activities?

4. Do you have any personal, cultural, or emotional hesitations about engaging with nature?

5. What local resources or community programs could help overcome these barriers?

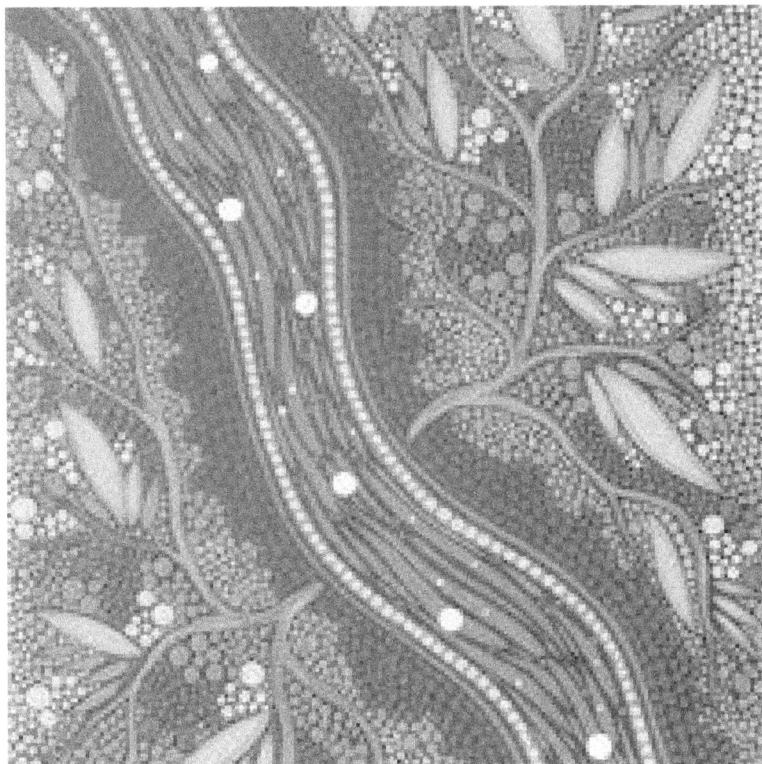

River Flow

Chapter 7

Expanding the Reach of Nature-Based Social Prescribing: Collaboration and Community Engagement

Overview:

This chapter focuses on the importance of collaboration and community engagement in expanding the reach of Nature-Based Social Prescribing (NBSP). By partnering with local environmental organizations, healthcare providers, community leaders, and government agencies, social workers can create a network of support that amplifies the impact of NBSP. The chapter also explores how community-based NBSP initiatives can contribute to larger environmental and social justice goals.

Key Topics:

7.1 Building Partnerships with Environmental Organizations

Local environmental organizations can be valuable partners in delivering NBSP programs. These organizations often have expertise in nature conservation, outdoor education, and community engagement, making them ideal collaborators in expanding access to nature-based interventions.

Strategies for Partnership Building:

- **Identify Key Stakeholders:** Social workers should start by identifying local environmental organizations, parks services, and outdoor activity groups that align with the goals of NBSP.

- **Collaborate on Program Delivery:** Partnering with environmental organizations allows for the co-creation of programs that benefit both clients and the local environment. For example, social workers might work with a conservation group to create a program where clients help restore local habitats as part of their NBSP plan.

- **Share Resources:** Environmental organizations often have access to outdoor spaces, equipment, and educational materials that can be used to support NBSP programs.

Example: A social worker partnered with a local conservation organization to create a weekly community gardening project for clients struggling with depression. In addition to benefiting the clients, the garden also served as a habitat restoration project for local wildlife.

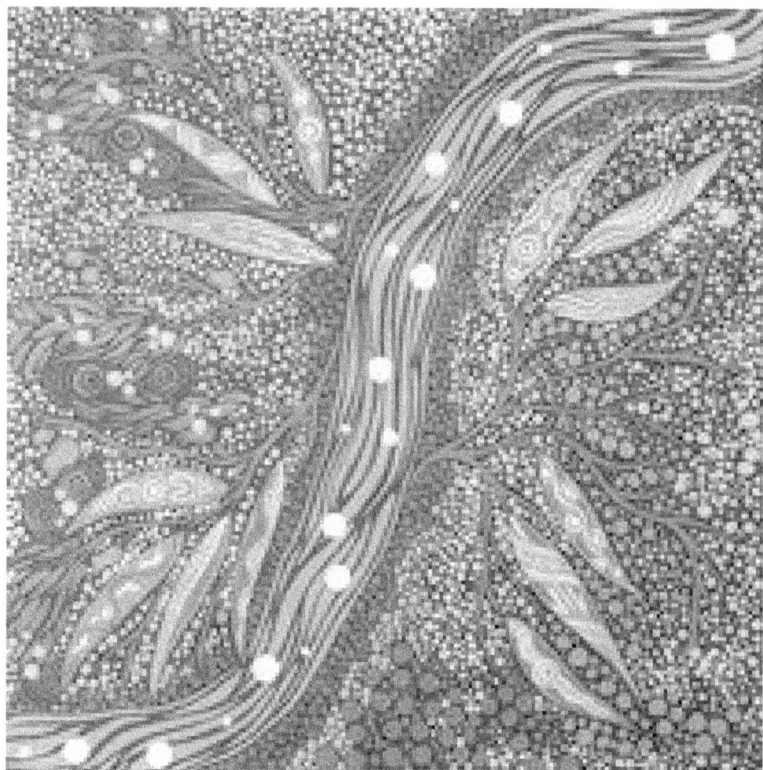

River

Chapter 8

Evaluating the Impact of Nature-Based Social Prescribing

Overview:

Evaluation is crucial to measure the effectiveness of Nature-Based Social Prescribing (NBSP) and to demonstrate its value to clients, stakeholders, and policymakers. This chapter focuses on how social workers can implement evaluation tools and methods to track progress, assess outcomes, and refine their approaches to NBSP interventions. It also highlights the importance of both qualitative and quantitative data to capture the holistic impact of nature-based interventions.

Key Topics:

8.1 Why Evaluation Matters in NBSP

Evaluating the outcomes of NBSP helps ensure that the prescribed interventions are beneficial and are tailored to each client's unique needs. Evaluation also provides evidence that can be used to advocate for wider implementation of NBSP in social work and healthcare settings. Effective evaluation supports continuous improvement, helping social workers refine their practices and ensure that they are meeting clients' physical, emotional, and social well-being.

Benefits of Evaluation:

- Demonstrates the effectiveness of NBSP to clients and stakeholders.

- Helps identify areas for improvement or modification in the intervention process.

- Provides a framework for documenting outcomes and success stories.

- Supports advocacy efforts by showing measurable results.

8.2 Types of Evaluation Methods

Evaluations can be qualitative (based on subjective feedback and observations) or quantitative (based on measurable data). A combination of both methods can offer a well-rounded view of the impact of NBSP.

Quantitative Methods:

- **Pre- and Post-Assessment Surveys:** These surveys can measure changes in clients' mood, stress levels, physical activity, and overall well-being before and after NBSP interventions. Standardized tools, such as the Warwick-Edinburgh Mental Well-being Scale (WEMWBS) or the Depression, Anxiety, and Stress Scales (DASS-21), can be useful for gathering quantitative data.

- **Tracking Physical Health:** For clients with health-related goals, measuring physical markers such as blood pressure, heart rate, or weight can show tangible improvements in physical health due to regular engagement with nature.

Qualitative Methods:

- **Client Self-Reports:** Regular check-ins and reflective journaling can allow clients to share how they feel emotionally and mentally before, during, and after their engagement with nature-based activities.

- **Focus Groups:** In group-based NBSP interventions, focus group discussions can provide valuable insights into how clients are experiencing the intervention and what changes they have noticed in their lives.

- **Observational Data:** Social workers can observe changes in clients' behaviour, mood, or engagement level during nature-based sessions. These observations can be combined with client self-reports for a fuller picture.

Example: After participating in a six-week NBSP program, clients were asked to complete the WEMWBS survey, which revealed a significant increase in overall well-being and a decrease in feelings of anxiety.

8.3 Creating Personalized Evaluation Tools

Each client's journey through NBSP will be unique, and social workers can create personalized evaluation tools that reflect the individual's goals and circumstances. Personalizing evaluation helps ensure that the measures used are relevant and meaningful for each client.

Steps for Creating Personalized Tools:

1. **Identify Client Goals:** At the start of the intervention, work with the client to identify specific goals (e.g., reducing stress, improving physical health, building social connections).

2. **Choose Relevant Measures:** Based on the client's goals, select specific quantitative or qualitative tools that will best capture progress. For example, a client

aiming to reduce stress might use a stress scale, while a client seeking social connection might complete a social engagement checklist.

3. **Track Progress Regularly:** Regular assessments—whether weekly, biweekly, or monthly—allow the client and social worker to track changes over time and adjust the intervention as needed.

Example: Tom, a client with high blood pressure, used a physical health log to track his blood pressure levels before and after each NBSP session. Over time, his levels improved, validating the positive impact of his engagement with nature.

8.4 Reporting Results to Stakeholders

For NBSP to gain broader acceptance and integration into healthcare systems, it is important to communicate the results of evaluations to key stakeholders, including healthcare providers, policymakers, community organizations, and funders. Clear, evidence-based reports can demonstrate the efficacy of NBSP and highlight its value to social, environmental, and healthcare outcomes.

Key Reporting Components:

- **Summary of Findings:** Include key data points that demonstrate improvements in clients' well-being, physical health, or social engagement. Use graphs, charts, or statistics to visually represent the data.

- **Case Studies:** Share individual success stories or case studies that illustrate the real-life impact of NBSP on clients' lives. Qualitative data such as testimonials or client reflections can bring the outcomes to life.

- **Recommendations:** Based on the evaluation, provide recommendations for future improvements or expansions of the NBSP program. Highlight areas where additional resources or support could further enhance client outcomes.

Example: A social worker shared a report with a local healthcare provider, showing that 80% of clients in the NBSP program reported a significant reduction in stress levels after six weeks of participation. This led to a pilot program integrating NBSP into the healthcare provider's treatment plans for clients with anxiety.

8.5 Continuous Improvement and Reflective Practice

Evaluation is not a one-time process but an ongoing part of delivering effective NBSP interventions. Continuous improvement involves regularly reviewing evaluation data, reflecting on what is working, and making necessary adjustments to enhance the client experience and maximize the benefits of nature-based interventions.

Tips for Continuous Improvement:

- **Regular Reflection:** After each NBSP session or at key points in the program, reflect on what went well and what could be improved. Discuss these reflections with clients, using their feedback to refine the intervention.

- **Adaptation to Client Needs:** As clients progress through NBSP, their needs may change. Be flexible in adapting the intervention to meet their evolving goals, whether that means shifting from physical activities to mindfulness-based practices or vice versa.

- **Stay Informed:** Keep up to date with the latest research and best practices in NBSP and related fields. By staying informed, social workers can ensure their interventions remain evidence-based and innovative.

Practical Tool: NBSP Evaluation Template

Use this template to evaluate the effectiveness of NBSP interventions with your clients. Modify the questions to suit individual client goals.

1. Client Information

    Name:

    Intervention Start Date:

    Primary Goals:

2. Pre-Assessment (Completed at the start of the intervention)

    a. How do you feel about your current level of physical, mental, and emotional well-being?

    b. What are your primary reasons for engaging in nature-based interventions?

3. Mid-Assessment (Completed halfway through the intervention)

    a. How would you rate your stress levels, mood, and physical health at this point?

    b. What changes have you noticed in your connection to nature?

4. Post-Assessment (Completed at the end of the intervention)

    a. Have your goals been met through this intervention? Please explain.

    b. Would you recommend nature-based interventions to others? Why or why not?

Chapter 9

Advocacy and Policy Development for Nature-Based Social Prescribing

Overview:

To fully realize the potential of Nature-Based Social Prescribing (NBSP), social workers must engage in advocacy and policy development. This chapter outlines how social workers can champion NBSP within their communities, influence policy decisions, and contribute to a broader movement of integrating nature-based interventions into mainstream healthcare and social services.

Key Topics:

9.1 The Role of Social Workers as Advocates

Social workers are uniquely positioned to advocate for policies that support the use of NBSP. By raising awareness about the mental, physical, and social benefits of nature-based interventions, social workers can influence policymakers, healthcare providers, and community leaders to adopt NBSP as a viable approach to improving well-being.

Advocacy Strategies:

- **Educating Policymakers:** Social workers can meet with local or national policymakers to discuss the importance of integrating NBSP into public health and social services. Presenting evidence of NBSP's effectiveness and sharing client success stories can make a compelling case for policy change.

- **Building Coalitions:** Partnering with environmental organizations, healthcare providers, and community groups can create a stronger, united voice for advocating for NBSP. Coalitions can amplify the message and push for policy changes at the local, state, or national level.

- **Public Awareness Campaigns:** Social workers can engage in public awareness campaigns to educate the broader community about NBSP and its benefits. This can involve writing articles, giving talks, or using social media platforms to spread the word.

Example: A group of social workers organized a community-wide campaign to advocate for green spaces in urban areas, leading to the creation of a new public park funded by local government.

9.2 Influencing Healthcare and Social Service Policies

For NBSP to be widely adopted, it must be formally recognized within healthcare and social service systems. Social workers can influence policy at the institutional level by advocating for NBSP programs to be included in treatment plans for mental health, chronic illness, and social isolation.

Steps to Influence Policy:

- **Presenting Research:** Social workers can present research findings on the benefits of NBSP to healthcare administrators and government agencies. Highlighting how NBSP can reduce healthcare costs, improve patient outcomes, and prevent burnout among caregivers can make a strong case for its integration into formal care plans.

- **Developing Policy Proposals:** Working with other stakeholders, social workers can draft policy proposals that outline the steps needed to implement NBSP at various levels of care. These proposals can address funding, program design, and training for social workers and healthcare providers on implementing nature-based interventions effectively.

9.3 Building Evidence for Policy Change

Gathering evidence is essential for effective advocacy. Social workers can compile data from evaluations, client feedback, and research studies to create a comprehensive picture of the effectiveness of NBSP. This evidence can be used to persuade stakeholders of the need for policy changes that support nature-based interventions.

Data Collection Strategies:

- **Case Studies and Testimonials:** Document case studies and client testimonials that highlight individual success stories and the transformative power of nature-based interventions. These narratives can serve as powerful tools in advocating for policy change.

- **Research Collaborations:** Partner with academic institutions or researchers to conduct studies on the outcomes of NBSP. Publishing peer-reviewed articles can enhance the credibility of NBSP and draw attention to its benefits in academic and policy-making circles.

- **Outcome Metrics:** Develop metrics to measure the impact of NBSP on various outcomes, including mental health, physical health, and social connectedness. Using standardized measures will allow for consistent data collection and comparison across different programs and settings.

Example: A social worker partnered with a university to conduct a longitudinal study on the impact of NBSP on depression rates among at-risk youth, leading to increased funding for nature-based programs in schools.

9.4 Engaging Community and Stakeholders

Engaging the community and stakeholders is vital for successful advocacy efforts. Social workers can mobilize support from clients, families, and local organizations to create a grassroots movement advocating for the adoption of NBSP.

Strategies for Community Engagement:

- **Community Meetings and Workshops:** Organize community meetings or workshops to discuss the benefits of NBSP and gather input from community members. Engaging clients and families in the conversation helps create a sense of ownership and investment in nature-based interventions.

- **Building Partnerships:** Form partnerships with local organizations, schools, and businesses to promote NBSP initiatives. Collaborative efforts can lead to resource sharing, funding opportunities, and increased visibility for nature-based programs.

- **Advocating for Inclusive Policies:** Ensure that advocacy efforts consider the needs of diverse populations, including marginalized communities. This involves promoting equitable access to nature-based resources and advocating for policies that address barriers to participation.

Example: A social worker organized a series of workshops in collaboration with local parks and recreation departments, leading to the establishment of free community nature walks tailored for individuals with mental health challenges.

9.5 Promoting Sustainability in Nature-Based Interventions

Advocacy for NBSP also involves promoting sustainable practices in the implementation of nature-based interventions. Ensuring that programs are ecologically sustainable will help protect the natural environments that clients engage with and foster a culture of environmental stewardship among participants.

Key Areas of Focus:

- **Environmental Education:** Incorporate educational components into NBSP that teach clients about local ecosystems, conservation efforts, and the importance of protecting nature. This awareness can encourage clients to become advocates for environmental sustainability themselves.

- **Sustainable Practices:** Advocate for practices within NBSP that minimize environmental impact, such as using local plants in garden-based activities or promoting low-impact outdoor activities. Emphasizing sustainability will not only enhance the experience of participants but also contribute to a healthier planet.

- **Community Green Initiatives:** Support and engage in local initiatives aimed at enhancing green spaces, such as tree planting events, community gardens, or conservation projects. These initiatives can foster community bonds while providing opportunities for clients to connect with nature.

Example: A social worker initiated a community garden project that engaged clients in planting and maintaining the garden, teaching them about sustainable gardening practices while providing therapeutic benefits.

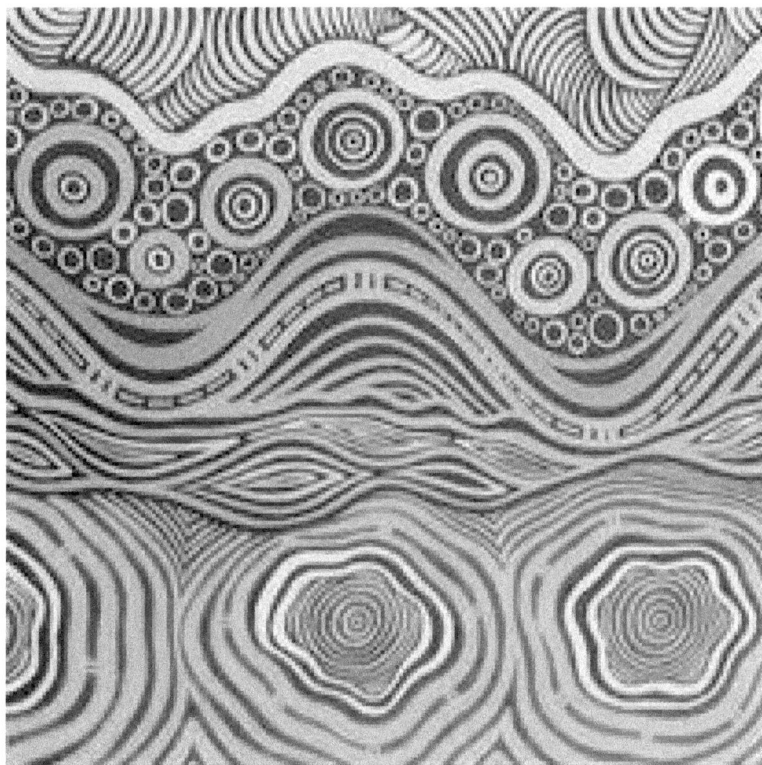

Rockpools

Chapter 10

Case Studies of Successful Nature-Based Social Prescribing Programs

Overview:

This chapter showcases real-world examples of successful Nature-Based Social Prescribing (NBSP) programs from various communities. By examining these case studies, social workers can gain insights into effective practices, challenges faced, and lessons learned in implementing NBSP.

Key Topics:

10.1 Case Study 1: Urban Nature Walks for Mental Health

In a metropolitan area, a social worker developed a program offering guided nature walks for individuals experiencing anxiety and depression. Participants engaged in mindfulness activities during walks, focusing on their surroundings and incorporating breathing exercises.

Outcomes:

- Participants reported reduced anxiety levels and improved mood.

- The program fostered a sense of community among participants, leading to continued friendships outside of walks.

Lessons Learned:

- Engaging local nature enthusiasts as volunteers enhanced the program's effectiveness.

- Incorporating mindfulness practices was crucial to the program's success.

10.2 Case Study 2: Community Gardening for Social Isolation

A rural community faced challenges related to social isolation, particularly among elderly residents. A social worker initiated a community gardening project where older adults could come together, grow vegetables, and share their gardening knowledge.

Outcomes:

- Participants reported increased social connections and a greater sense of belonging.

- The project provided fresh produce, improving nutritional intake among participants.

Lessons Learned:

- Partnerships with local agriculture organizations helped provide resources and expertise.

- Addressing mobility challenges by creating accessible gardening options was vital for participation.

10.3 Case Study 3: Therapeutic Nature-Based Retreats for Trauma Recovery

A non-profit organization in a suburban area developed therapeutic retreats that combined nature-based activities with trauma-informed care for individuals recovering from PTSD. Participants engaged in activities such as hiking, yoga, and nature journaling.

Outcomes:

- Participants experienced a significant reduction in PTSD symptoms, with many reporting improved coping skills.

- Feedback indicated that the serene environment of nature facilitated deeper emotional processing.

Lessons Learned:

- Creating a safe, trauma-informed environment was essential for client comfort.

- Integrating experienced facilitators trained in trauma care improved the quality of the retreats.

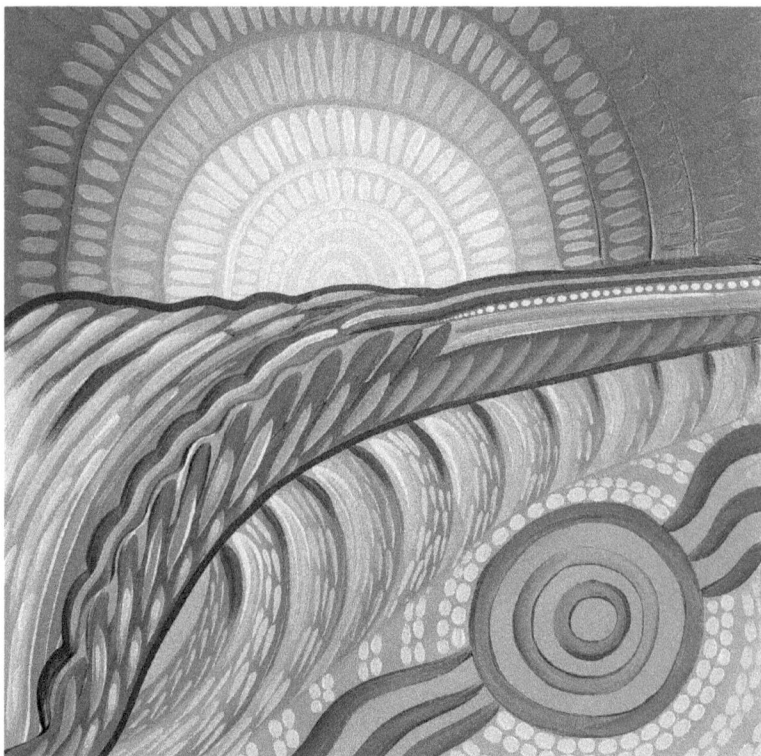

Salt Water Connection

Chapter 11

Future Directions for Nature-Based Social Prescribing

Emerging Trends in Nature-Based Social Prescribing

As the field of social work continues to evolve, Nature-Based Social Prescribing (NBSP) is gaining momentum as an innovative approach to promoting well-being. This chapter explores emerging trends, potential future developments, and recommendations for integrating nature-based interventions into social work practice.

1. Integration of Technology

With the rise of digital technology, there is an increasing opportunity to integrate tech solutions into nature-based interventions. Apps and online platforms can facilitate connections between clients and local nature resources, provide information on outdoor activities, and support community engagement. For instance, mobile applications that encourage nature exploration through gamification or social networking can enhance client motivation and participation.

2. Personalized Nature Experiences

The future of NBSP may include more personalized nature experiences tailored to individual preferences, needs, and cultural backgrounds. Utilizing assessments to understand clients' unique connections to nature and their interests can help social workers design interventions that resonate deeply with clients. This personalized approach fosters greater engagement and satisfaction.

3. Collaboration with Health Care Providers

As the evidence supporting the benefits of nature-based interventions grows, social workers may find increased collaboration with healthcare providers. Integrating NBSP into holistic healthcare models, such as primary care and mental health services, can create a comprehensive approach to well-being. This collaboration allows for a more interdisciplinary approach, where social workers, therapists, and healthcare providers work together to enhance clients' mental, emotional, and physical health.

4. Incorporation of Indigenous Knowledge

Increasing recognition of the value of Indigenous knowledge in understanding and engaging with nature can inform future practices in NBSP. By incorporating traditional ecological knowledge and practices, social workers can create more culturally relevant interventions that respect Indigenous perspectives and strengthen community ties. Collaborating with Indigenous communities can provide valuable insights into sustainable practices and holistic well-being.

5. Focus on Environmental Sustainability

As the climate crisis escalates, there is a growing awareness of the interconnectedness of social and environmental well-being. Future nature-based social prescribing initiatives may focus more on environmental sustainability and conservation, encouraging clients to engage in activities that promote ecological stewardship. This dual focus can enhance clients' sense of purpose while contributing to community well-being.

Research and Evidence Base

Continued research is essential for establishing a robust evidence base for nature-based interventions. Future directions for research may include:

1. Longitudinal Studies

Conducting longitudinal studies to examine the long-term impacts of NBSP on mental health, social connections, and overall well-being will provide valuable insights into the sustainability of benefits over time.

2. Diverse Populations

Expanding research to include diverse populations, such as individuals with disabilities, marginalized communities, and various age groups, can help understand the unique needs and outcomes of different client groups.

3. Exploring Mechanisms of Change

Investigating the mechanisms by which nature-based interventions impact well-being will deepen our understanding of how these practices work. Research can explore physiological, psychological, and social processes that contribute to positive outcomes, informing practice and policy.

Recommendations for Social Workers

As nature-based social prescribing continues to evolve, social workers can take proactive steps to enhance their practice:

1. Stay Informed and Engage in Professional Development

Keep abreast of emerging trends, research findings, and best practices in NBSP through professional development opportunities, conferences, and workshops. Engaging with the broader community of practice can foster innovation and collaboration.

2. Advocate for Nature-Based Interventions

Advocate for the inclusion of nature-based interventions in social work policy and practice. Share success stories, research findings, and the benefits of NBSP with stakeholders to promote support for these initiatives within organizations and communities.

3. Foster Community Partnerships

Build partnerships with local organizations, environmental groups, and healthcare providers to create collaborative networks that support nature-based programs. Engaging community stakeholders enhances resources and amplifies the impact of interventions.

4. Engage in Reflective Practice

Continuously reflect on your experiences and the effectiveness of nature-based interventions. Seek feedback from clients and colleagues, and be open to adapting practices based on lessons learned and new insights.

5. Promote Equity and Inclusion

Prioritize equity and inclusion in nature-based social prescribing initiatives. Ensure that programs are accessible and culturally relevant for all clients, and actively work to address systemic barriers to participation.

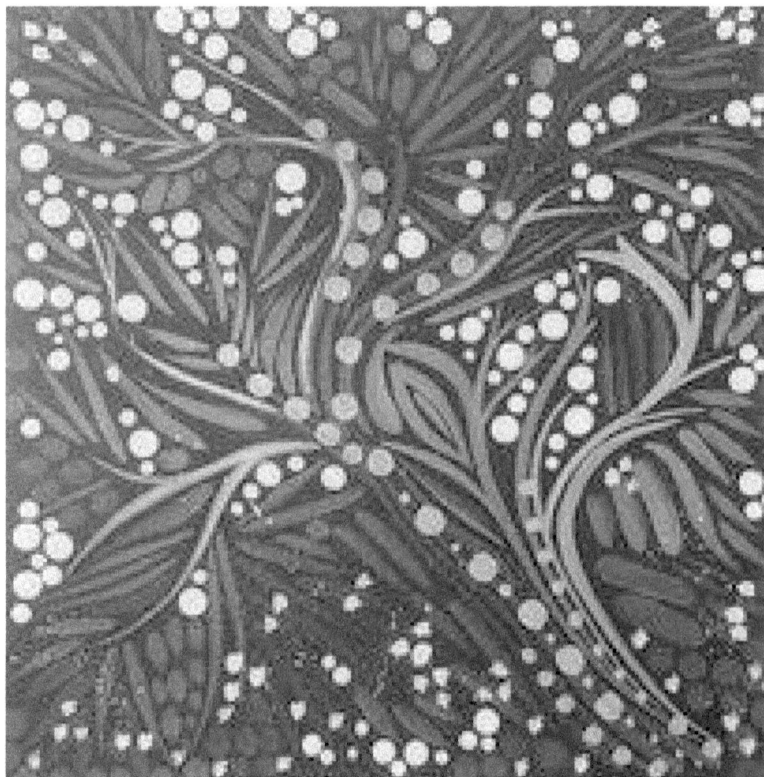

Wattle 2

Conclusion

The future of Nature-Based Social Prescribing holds immense potential for promoting holistic well-being. By embracing emerging trends, conducting rigorous research, and fostering community collaboration, social workers can enhance their practice and contribute to a more sustainable and equitable society. As we move forward, the integration of nature-based interventions offers a powerful opportunity to connect individuals with nature, each other, and themselves, ultimately enriching the social work profession and the communities it serves.

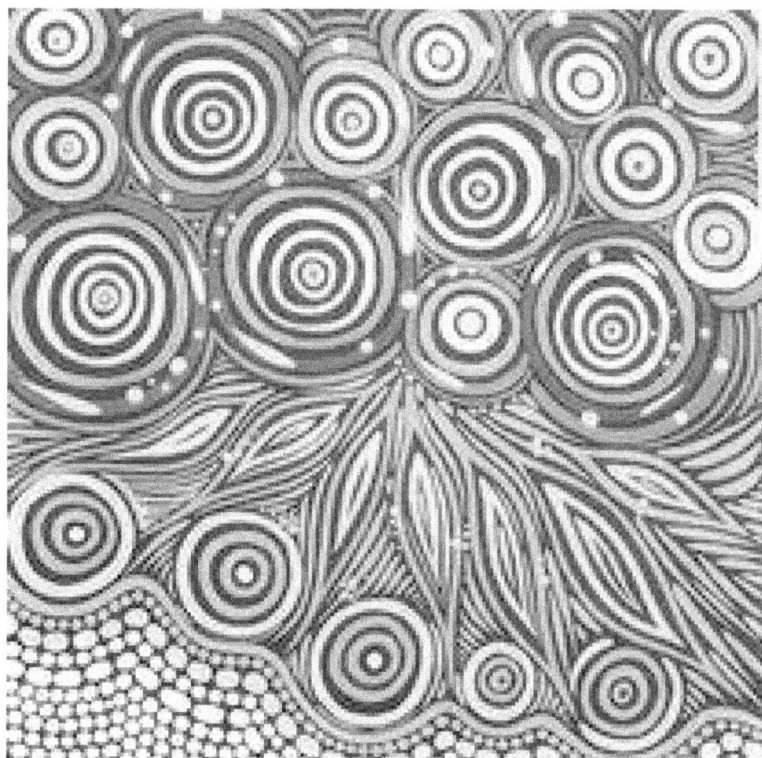

Wattle

Reference List

Berman, M. G., Jonides, J., & Kaplan, S. (2008). "The cognitive benefits of interacting with nature." Psychological Science, 19(12), 1207-1212.

Bratman, G. N., Daily, G. C., Levy, B. J., & Gross, J. J. (2015). "The benefits of nature experience: Improved affect and cognition." Trends in Cognitive Sciences, 19(12), 841-849.

Chawla, L. (2015). "Benefits of Nature Contact for Children." Journal of Planning Literature, 30(4), 433-452.

Cohen-Cline, H., Turkheimer, E., & Duncan, G. E. (2015). "Access to green space, physical activity, and mental health: a twin study." Journal of Epidemiology & Community Health, 69(6), 523-529.

Frumkin, H., Bratman, G. N., Breslow, S. J., Cochran, B., Kahn, P. H., Lawler, J. J., Levin, P. S., Tandon, P. S., Varanasi, U., Wolf, K. L., & Wood, S. A. (2017). "Nature Contact and Human Health: A Research Agenda." Environmental Health Perspectives, 125(7), 075001.

Gonzalez, M. T., Hartig, T., Patil, G. G., Martinsen, E. W., & Kirkevold, M. (2010). "Therapeutic horticulture in clinical depression: A prospective study." Research and Theory for Nursing Practice, 24(4), 227-241.

Holt-Lunstad, J., Smith, T. B., & Layton, J. B. (2010). "Social relationships and mortality risk: A meta-analytic review." PLoS Medicine, 7(7), e1000316.

Jordan, M., & Hinds, J. (2016). Ecotherapy: Theory, Research and Practice. Macmillan International Higher Education.

Kaplan, S. (1995). "The restorative benefits of nature: Toward an integrative framework." Journal of Environmental Psychology, 15(3), 169-182.

Li, Q. (2010). "Effect of forest bathing trips on human immune function." Environmental Health and Preventive Medicine, 15(1), 9-17.

Maller, C., Townsend, M., Pryor, A., Brown, P., & St Leger, L. (2006). "Healthy nature healthy people: 'Contact with nature' as an upstream health promotion intervention for populations." Health Promotion International, 21(1), 45-54.

Marselle, M. R., Irvine, K. N., & Warber, S. L. (2014). "Examining Group Walks in Nature and Multiple Aspects of Well-Being: A Large-Scale Study." Ecopsychology, 6(3), 134-147.

Martyn, P., & Brymer, E. (2016). "The relationship between nature relatedness and anxiety." Journal of Health Psychology, 21(7), 1436-1445.

Natural England. (2016). "A Review of Nature-Based Interventions for Mental Health Care." Natural England Commissioned Report NECR204.

Pretty, J., Peacock, J., Sellens, M., & Griffin, M. (2005). "The mental and physical health outcomes of green exercise." International Journal of Environmental Health Research, 15(5), 319-337.

Richardson, M., & Sheffield, D. (2017). "Three good things in nature: Noticing nearby nature brings sustained increases in connection with nature." Ecopsychology, 9(4), 231-241.

Rogerson, M., Barton, J., Bragg, R., & Pretty, J. (2017). "The health and well-being impacts of volunteering with The Conservation Volunteers: A review." The Conservation Volunteers & University of Essex.

Sempik, J., Hine, R., & Wilcox, D. (Eds.). (2010). Green Care: A Conceptual Framework. Loughborough University Centre for Child and Family Research.

Ulrich, R. S. (1984). "View through a window may influence recovery from surgery." Science, 224(4647), 420-421.

Williams, F., & Lenton, A. P. (2007). "The power of the first impression: Do first impressions based on static facial appearance affect dynamic impressions?" British Journal of Social Psychology, 46(4), 587-598.

World Health Organization (WHO). (2016). "Urban green spaces and health: A review of evidence." WHO Regional Office for Europe.

Additional Resources

1. **Nature-Based Therapy**
   (www.naturebasedtherapy.com.au)
   A comprehensive resource providing insights, training, and services related to nature-based therapeutic practices. It offers educational tools and programs designed for professionals, including social workers, therapists, and educators, focusing on integrating nature-based therapy into various settings.

Recommended Reading

"Braiding Sweetgrass: Indigenous Wisdom, Scientific Knowledge, and the Teachings of Plants" by Robin Wall Kimmerer

> This beloved book combines Indigenous wisdom with botanical science. Kimmerer, a member of the Citizen Potawatomi Nation, offers a poetic and profound exploration of the natural world, emphasizing reciprocal relationships with plants and the land.

"Sand Talk: How Indigenous Thinking Can Save the World" by Tyson Yunkaporta

> Yunkaporta, an Indigenous Australian, presents a fascinating perspective on sustainable living and interconnectedness. He uses Indigenous wisdom and symbolism to discuss complex societal and environmental challenges.

"Phosphorescence: On Awe, Wonder and Things That Sustain You When the World Goes Dark" by Julia Baird

> This reflective memoir explores the healing power of nature, awe, and resilience. Baird shares her journey of finding light in dark times through her connection to the ocean, natural beauty, and quiet moments.

"The Nature Fix: Why Nature Makes Us Happier, Healthier, and More Creative" by Florence Williams

This book examines the science behind the benefits of spending time in nature, from stress relief to improved creativity. Williams provides an engaging, research-backed look at how nature positively impacts well-being.

"Belonging: Remembering Ourselves Home"
by Toko-pa Turner

Turner draws from her background in Jungian psychology, dreamwork, and Indigenous wisdom to explore the themes of belonging and connection to the earth. Her work emphasizes reclaiming lost connections to community and nature.

"Lost Connections: Uncovering the Real Causes of Depression – and the Unexpected Solutions" by Johann Hari

Hari delves into the broader social and environmental factors that contribute to mental health challenges, exploring how connection—to nature, people, and purpose—plays a crucial role in healing and well-being.

"Gathering Moss: A Natural and Cultural History of Mosses" by Robin Wall Kimmerer

Another beautiful work by Kimmerer, this book reveals the tiny but intricate world of mosses and invites readers to consider how these small plants offer wisdom about resilience, community, and interconnectedness.

"Forest Bathing: How Trees Can Help You Find Health and Happiness" by Dr. Qing Li

Dr. Li, a leading researcher on forest therapy, explains the health benefits of spending time in nature, particularly in forests. This book provides practical insights and scientific research on the Japanese practice of "Shinrin-yoku" or forest bathing.

"The Secret Wisdom of Nature: Trees, Animals, and the Extraordinary Balance of All Living Things" by Peter Wohlleben

Wohlleben explores the delicate relationships and symbiotic connections in nature, advocating for a more respectful and harmonious relationship with the environment.

"Original Instructions: Indigenous Teachings for a Sustainable Future" edited by Melissa K. Nelson

This anthology gathers essays from Indigenous thinkers and activists who share their traditional ecological knowledge and philosophies on environmental stewardship, health, and sustainability.

www.ingramcontent.com/pod-product-compliance
Lightning Source LLC
Chambersburg PA
CBHW051248020426
42333CB00025B/3109